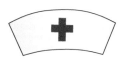

THIS BOOK BELONGS
TO A FUTURE NURSE

_____

GIVEN ON

_____

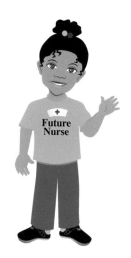

The Adventures of Nurse Nicole

Educating the World Through the Art & Science of Nursing

Written by Nicole M. Brown
Illustrated by Francine Smith

www.nursenicole.co

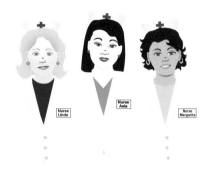

Nurses are Blessed!

This book is dedicated to nurses everywhere, current nursing students, the next generation of nurses to come, everyone who has been cared for by a nurse, and to my children Nathaniel, Nicolas, and Nicola.

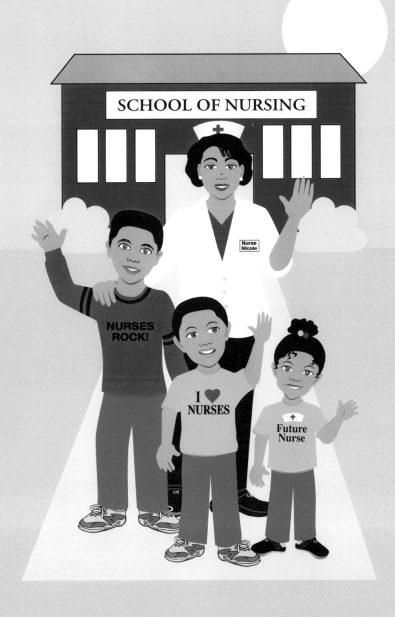

Grandpa drops Nate, Nick and Nicola off at their Mom's job, the Nursing School. They hug their Mom and wave goodbye to Grandpa.

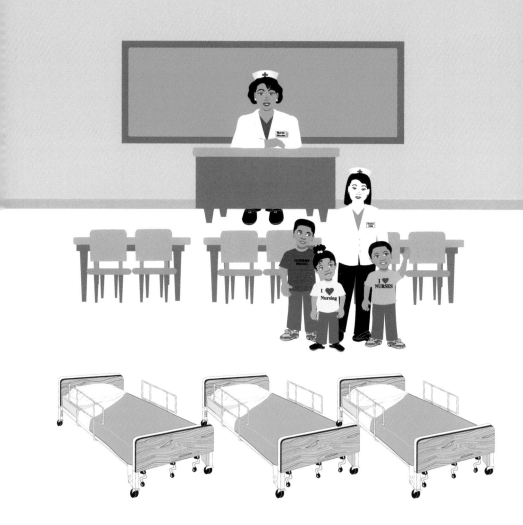

Nicola asks,
"What do you do at work Mom?"
Nate asks, "Are you a dentist?"
Nick asks, "Are you a doctor?"

Mom replies,
"At work I'm Nurse Nicole,
I am a nurse who teaches nursing."
A nurse helps people who are sick.

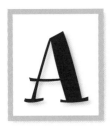

is for **Ambulance**.
A nurse helps people who ride to the hospital in an ambulance.

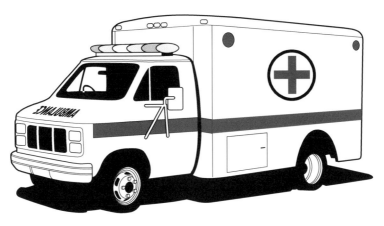

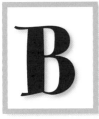

is for **Bedside Table**.
A nurse helps people eat meals from their bedside table when they need help.

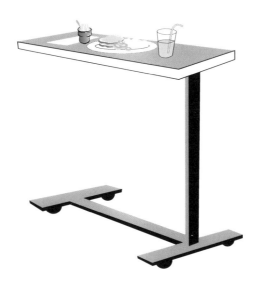

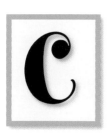

is for **Call Light**.
A nurse makes sure the call light is within a
patient's reach so they can call for help.

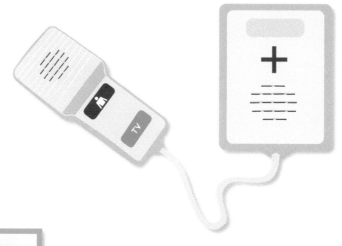

is for **Doctor.**
A doctor and a nurse work together to help
the patient feel better.

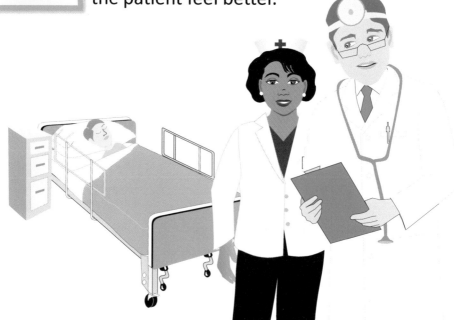

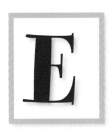

is for **Equipment.**
A nurse uses equipment like tongue blades and cotton balls to help people who are sick.

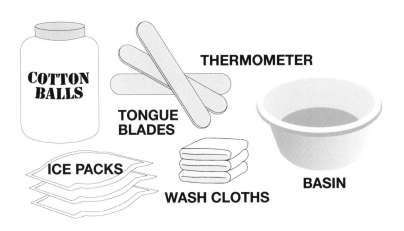

COTTON BALLS

THERMOMETER

TONGUE BLADES

ICE PACKS

WASH CLOTHS

BASIN

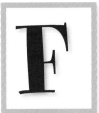

is for **Family.**
A nurse calms the family by explaining procedures to them.

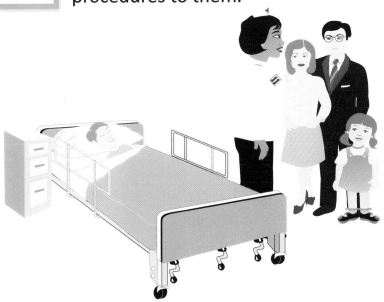

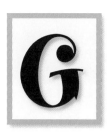

is for **Gloves.**
A nurse wears gloves to prevent the spread of germs.

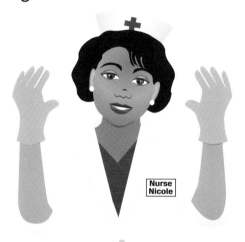

Nurse
Nicole

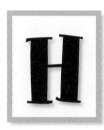

is for **Hospital.**
A nurse helps people who go to the hospital because they are sick or need an operation.

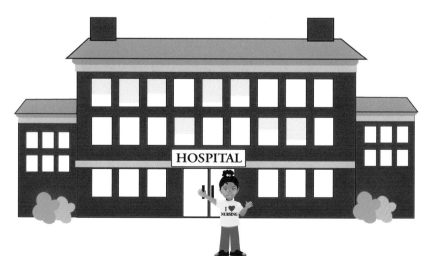

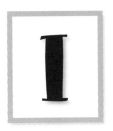

I is for **Illness.**
A nurse helps people get better who suffer from an illness.

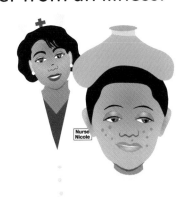

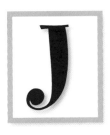

J is for **Joint.**
A nurse helps people move their knee joint after surgery or an injury.

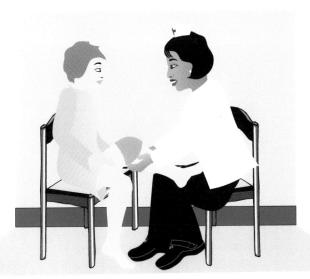

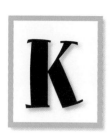

K is for **Kerlix.**
A nurse uses a kerlix bandage to cover a wound.

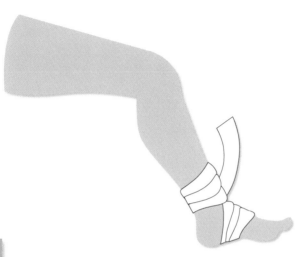

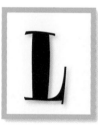

L is for **Love.**
A nurse likes helping people.
They love what they do!

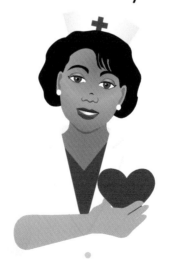

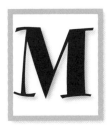

is for **Medicine.**
A nurse gives people medicine to make them feel better.

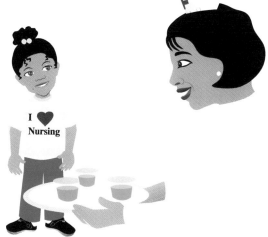

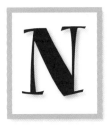

is for **Nurse.**
A nurse is a person who takes care of people who are sick in the hospital.

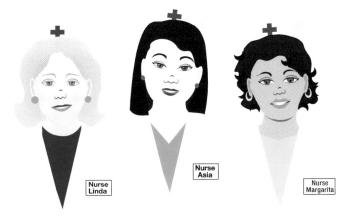

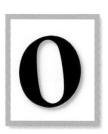

is for **Operation.**
A nurse prepares a patient for an operation
and helps during a procedure.

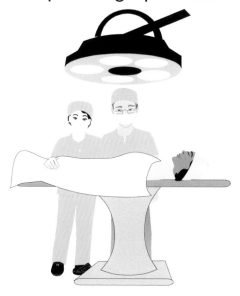

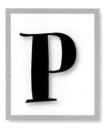

is for **Patient.**
Patients are people who are sick in the
hospital. A nurse helps patients get better.

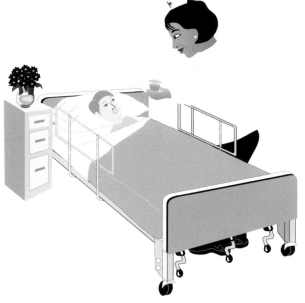

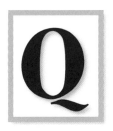

is for **Question.**
A nurse asks and answers questions to
help people understand their condition.

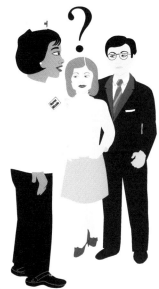

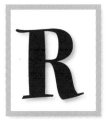

is for **Room.**
A nurse helps people to their room
after they are admitted to the hospital.

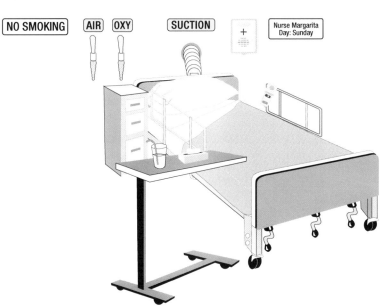

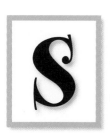

S is for **Stethescope.**
A nurse uses a stethescope to listen to a person's heart and lungs when they are sick.

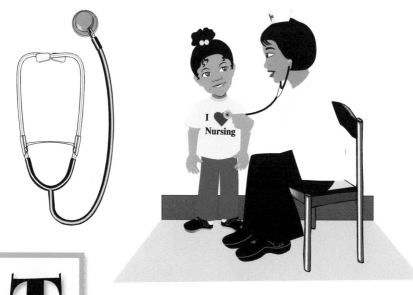

T is for **Thermometer.**
A nurse uses a thermometer to check a person's temperature for a fever.

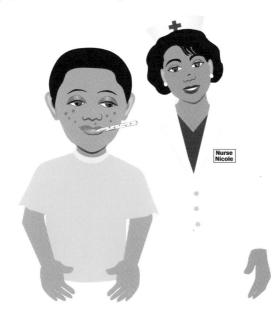

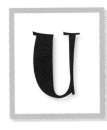

is for **Uniform.**
A nurse wears a uniform and sometimes a cap when helping people in the hospital.

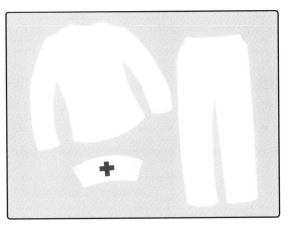

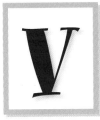

is for **Vital** signs.
Vital signs are pulse, temperature, blood pressure, and respirations. Nurses check vital signs when people are sick and well.

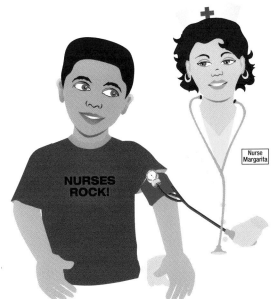

NURSES
ROCK!

Nurse
Margarita

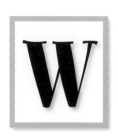

is for **Wheelchair.**
A nurse uses a wheelchair to move patients from place to place in the hospital.

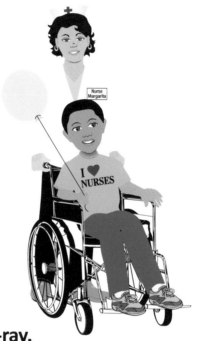

is for **X-ray.**
A nurse uses X-rays to see if a bone is broken or where the pain is located.

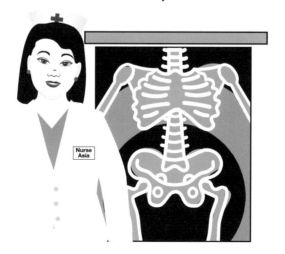

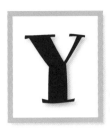

is for **Yearly.**
A nurse reminds people when its time for their yearly physical check up.

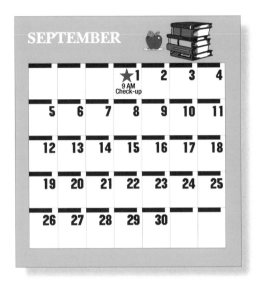

SEPTEMBER

			★1 9 AM Check-up	2	3	4
5	6	7	8	9	10	11
12	13	14	15	16	17	18
19	20	21	22	23	24	25
26	27	28	29	30		

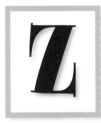

is for **Zinc.**
Zinc is a medicine used to help people feel better.

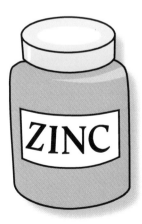

ZINC

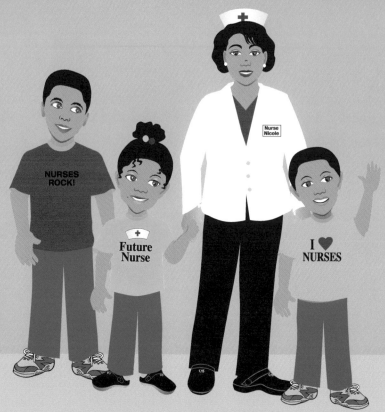

"You see by using the letters of the alphabet
I've shown you just how nurses help people.
I hope one day you will want to be
a nurse like me."

Nicola says,
"I want to help people when I grow up."
Nate asks,
"Is nursing only for girls?"
Nick asks,
"Can boys be nurses too?"

Nurse Nicole says,
"The profession of nursing is open to everyone!
Always remember
N is for Nurse!"

NURSE NICOLE QUIZ

1. What does Nurse Nicole do?

2. Where does Nurse Nicole work?

3. Who came to visit Nurse Nicole?

4. Who do nurses take care of?

5. Do you want to be a nurse?

6. What did you like about nursing?

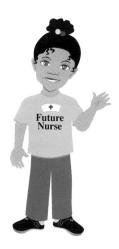

7. What does the letter A stand for?

   a. apple

   b. apron

   c. ambulance

8. What does the letter H stand for?

   a. hospital

   b. health

   c. head

9. Why do nurses take a temperature?

   a. check for a stomach ache

   b. check for a fever

   c. check your heart rate

10. What equipment do nurses use?

   a. cotton balls

   b. ice packs

   c. tongue blades

   d. wash cloths

   e. all the above

11. What do nurses wear to prevent infection?

12. What kind of bandage covers wounds?

13. What do nurses use to listen to heart and lung sounds?

14. What do nurses wear while working?

15. What do nurses use to move patients from room-to-room?

16. When should people get their wellness check-up?

THE ADVENTURES OF NURSE NICOLE

Educating the World Through the Art & Science of Nursing

N is for NURSE

By Nicole M. Brown

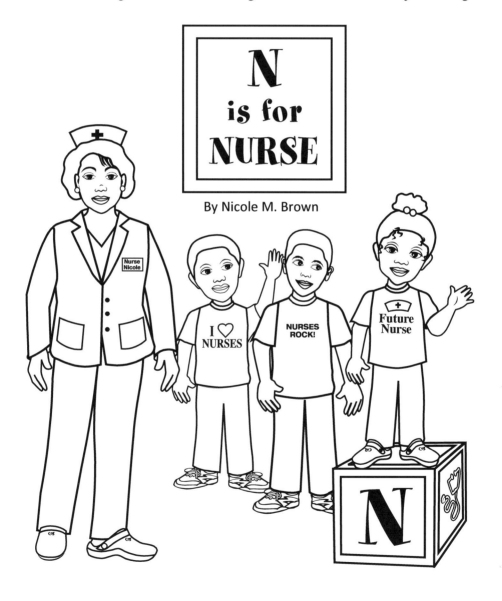

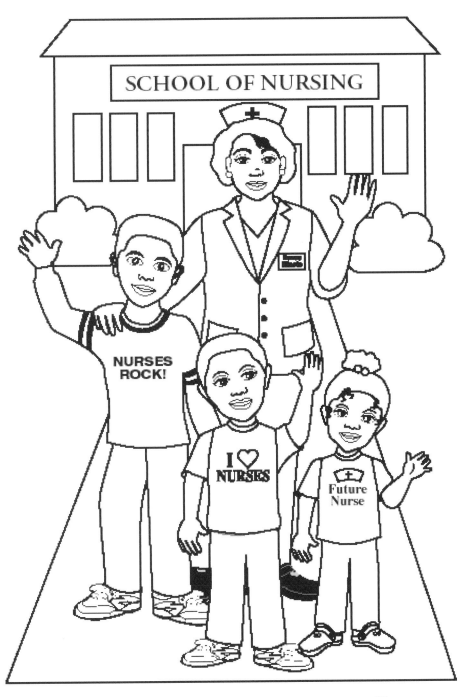

Color us "Future Nurses."

CPSIA information can be obtained at www.ICGtesting.com
Printed in the USA
LVIW01n2019080118
562247LV00001B/27